The Smart way to lose Weight. Rapid Weight loss using a Sex Diet!

By **Sean Parker**

Text

Since the beginning of time, humans have made love, fallen in love played protected and nurtured one another. And I'd often wonder which is the most powerful aspect of human nature, love or sex. Love compared to sexual satisfaction and not for reproductive purposes, but simply for sexual pleasure, the pursuit of sexual satisfaction is one of the most powerful emotions we have and share with one another. But what if we can tap into our overwhelming desire for sexual satisfaction and hardwire our brain for weight loss. I was 410lbs and miserable, I tried every diet out there, and I mean every diet, but nothing seemed to work for me. One day I was walking on the Levee, headed towards the Algiers ferry, I'm from Marrero Louisiana the west bank side of New Orleans, and I'd go walking on top the newly paved Levee.

A beautiful place to walk for exercise,

for miles and miles it's just evenly paved

walkway, I'd just park my car two and a

half miles away from the Algiers ferry,

and I'd walk to the ferry, take a 30-

minute break and walk back to my car, a

5 mile walk every day, I looked at losing

weight like fighting a war, I guess a war

against obesity, or maybe against my

own laziness. But one day, as I made it

back to my car, on a particular grueling

hot summer's day, I was dripping from sweat head to toe, as I approached my car, there was an older gentleman exiting his car, "hot day young man" he said. "Yes sir, it's burning up out here, but at least it gives me a chance to sweat off some of this weigh." I said. "I lost 390lbs and I didn't even break a sweat, not once!" he said. "What! How did you do that?" I asked. "A year ago, I lost my wife of 40 years to cancer,

devastated and heartbroken, alone and
by myself, confused and a little
depressed, I guess, emotionally I
completely shut down, and just stop
eating, I lost my appetite and began to
lose weight rapidly, oh, I'd eat enough
to sustain myself, but with my wife
gone, going out to dinner and home
cooked meals and family dinners
seemed pointless without my wife, so I
became sort of a recluse, just staying

home but losing weight from being sad. Until one day I just picked myself up and realized my wife wouldn't want me wasting away like this, (if she were here, she would say stop feeling sorry for yourself and live your life!) And that's just what I did, I started going out again, at first a little bit, but gradually more and more, meeting new people developing new interest and enjoying my life again, that's why I'm here at the park today, I'm glad I bumped into you

and we had a chance to talk young man.

I lost 390lbs in 9 months just staying

inside finding myself! So, you don't

necessarily have to work so hard to lose

weight, I just cut back on eating and the

weight just fell off me!" he said. I shook

the nice old guy hand, and thanked him

for his advice, I got into my car and head

for home, thinking about what the man

had said me, about controlling what you

eat, and then I had an idea just pop into my head, what if I could change my desire for food to a desire for sexual satisfaction?! What if every time I get hungry instead I get horny, instead of eating for pleasure I could have sex for pleasure, for go food and seek instead more and more intense orgasm's, eating only enough to sustain my body, like the old man did! The next day I designed a radical new diet program for myself, something to test my determination to walk 5 miles every day, combined with a search for dramatic results, remember I've been walking 5 miles every day for 6 months, and I haven't had any significant weight loss, a pound or two here and there but I couldn't keep the weight off, I'd lose 3 pounds and then gain 2 pounds back in a day or two, but no real significant change in my weight loss, I started at 410lbs and after 6 months I still weighed 400lbs, so, I decided to make a tactical change to my diet plan, no more 5 mile walks for me, I'll approach my weakness for food, by transforming my appetite for eating, into instant gratification for sexual satisfaction, buy training my brain to crave sex instead of food, I'd have an orgasm to replace the feeling of being hungry, I calculated how many times I'd get hungry in a day, verse how many times I'd get horny in a day, and it

wasn't even close, from personal

observation I'd get hungry 4 to 5 times a

day, once in the morning, once midday

about 12o'clock and once in the evening

about 7 or 8 o'clock and once more

before I'd go to bed at night, and that

was it! However, it pales in comparison,

to how many times a day I'd think about

sex, it starts even before the day does,

in the form of erotic dreams, I often

wake up 4 to 5 a.m. in the morning, being disturbed from a sound sleep with erotic images flashing in my mind, like some homemade porn movie or something. All I know is, it wakes me up feeling extremely horny and I can't get back to sleep without an orgasm. Even during my early morning ritual of brushing my teeth washing my face, trimming my beard, and constantly thought-out the day, if I had to tally an exact number, I'd say out of a 24-hour period, I thought about sex every 35 seconds! And with that revelation, I realized that sex was the key to controlling my insatiable appetite for food, from my own inward looking personal research, it was clear to me, I'd much rather be having sex then eating so much food, so, I decided to eat one meal every other day, and explore my appetite for sexual escapades on the days I don't eat. So, I can eat one meal on Monday but nothing on Tuesday, I can eat one meal on Wednesday but nothing on Thursday, and again one meal on Friday but nothing on Saturday, and one meal on Sunday, and on and on. Until I see some results, but I wouldn't have to wait long, because that first week I lost 15lbs, I couldn't believe what my scale was reading! I always weigh myself first thing in the morning, without clothing, and at the same time every morning, and record the results, and there was no comparison, the results from this new diet plan was outstanding! On the days I can eat, I try to eat about 12 o'clock p.m. but no later than 3 o'clock p.m. and I'm not hungry the entire day, because just when I get hungry at work around 10 o'clock a.m. it's close to launch time, and after I have eaten for launch time, I'm usually satisfied and full the entire day, and since I only eat one time a day, I can choose to eat whatever I wanted too, barbecue ribs with steak fries, jambalaya, or red beans and rice, seafood gumbo, boiled crawfish and crabs, or fried catfish, stuffed bell peppers lasagna, baked macaroni and cheese and dirty rice. I know, but I'm from the south and we eat down here, ask anybody, we love food! And it's so delicious and almost impossible to resist and I haven't even started on the delicacies for dessert! But on the day's, I don't eat, I focus my attentions on sexual satisfaction instead of instant gratification, that I would normally get from eating food, every time I got hungry I'd make love to my fiancée, and without her love, support and encouragement, none of this would be possible. In fact, she was the one who suggested that I get active and lose weight, and I'm so thankful for her being in my life, because this diet is not for the faint of heart, it takes dedication, self-reliance determination and the unmitigated gall, to believe you can achieve the impossible and take control of your own life, with this diet you have the ability to reshape your body. My toughest challenge was the first week, and the most grueling was the first day without eating any food, it

"SUCKED!" Going 24 hours without

eating anything, I was irritable I felt

week and frustrated, but I stuck to my

guns and I toughed it out. The next day I

woke up, and I felt fine in fact I wasn't

even hungry, until about 10:00 a.m. my

hunger pain kick in, and I had launch at

12 o'clock p.m. well, I had a great big

launch, I was full and satisfied the entire

day, next day was much easier to get

through the 24 hours without eating, every time I thought about food, I would put that thought out of my mind by thinking about sex, and if thinking about sex wasn't persuasive enough to alter my thought patterns, I would have to achieve a physical orgasm, to make me stop thinking about eating food. And it works, time after time, the pleasure from sex is a far greater human experience, then tasting food. And the more I craved sex the less I craved food.

About the third day into this new diet is

when I had a major breakthrough, my

cravings for food dropped significantly,

and when I did eat, my portions were

smaller on my dinner plate, because I

was eating less food my stomach shrink

in size, and I didn't need to eat as much

food to fill full, I begin saving so much

money, I couldn't believe it, all the extra

money that went on fast food, was

adding up to quite a bit of money, which

lead me to conclude, I was spending

23% of my income on food, that

realization was amazing for me! Not

only I am losing weight fast but I'm

saving money too! This seems unreal,

except for the fact I can't eat anything

for 24-hours, don't get me wrong, I'm

grateful I found a real solution to lose

weight, but it's not easy, my temptation

has lessened over time, but it still exists,

and I must admit it's easier to control

my appetite, than walk 5 miles every

day. I'd lose a steady 5 to 10 pounds

every week depending if I cheated on

my diet, let's face it, we all do it, we all

cheat on our diet, even if just a little bit,

but my main focus was always to be as

strict and rigid as possible to achieve the

best results. I started at 400lbs and lost

an average of 5lbs a week, over the next

6 months I lost 120lbs, and it felt great

losing all that weight, my stamina was
through the roof, my blood pressure
was in check, my clothes were falling off
me, and I had some nice clothes for a
big guy, I could no longer fit some of my
favorite clothes, and that sucked, I
guess a small price to pay, for such
awesome results. Now standing at 6'1
280lbs and I feel the best I have every
felt in my life! Over the next 2 months I
lose another 60lbs and my weight stays

a steady 220lbs, which is my dream size,

now that I've achieved my goal, my new

battle is to maintain my body weight.

I'm sitting down to write this in hopes of

inspiring others to find their own

pathway, to lose weight successfully.

My journey was uniquely mine, but my

hope is that you as individuals find your

own pathway to happiness and

successful weight loss with your own

uniquely designed diet program.

GOOD LUCK OUT THERE AND GOD BLESS!